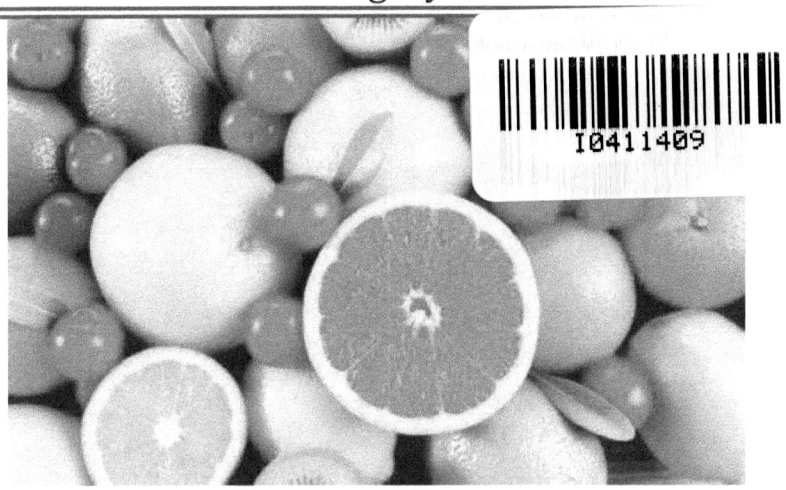

My Personal Journey Through Bariatric Surgery

Sophia Frazier

My Personal Journey Through Bariatric Surgery

My Personal Journey Through Bariatric Surgery

I wrote this book for others who might be considering making the commitment to healthier living. Bariatric procedures are not for everyone. Keep in mind that this should be considered a permanent procedure to use as a tool to make lifestyle changes possible for those of us who have difficulty maintaining a healthy weight any other way.

It should be considered as a last resort after all other methods have been tried. Please obtain the advice of a physician before beginning any regimen or procedure that could affect your health and your life.

Each center for bariatric weight loss will have its own specific guidelines. Keep in mind that mine are specifically from St. Vincent Bariatric Weight Loss Center of Excellence based in Carmel, Indiana. Your guidelines may be different. Please follow your physician's orders.

Also, be aware that if you have an addictive personality then you may be tempted to substitute the addiction to food with another addiction. Seek professional advice when needed.

The information in this book, by no means should be substituted for professional help. Investigate and research the options that are best for you. Seek the advice of a physician. This is indeed my personal journey and I hope that the information within gives the reader more awareness regarding bariatric surgery. And by all means, GOOD LUCK

.---Sophia Frazier

My Personal Journey Through Bariatric Surgery

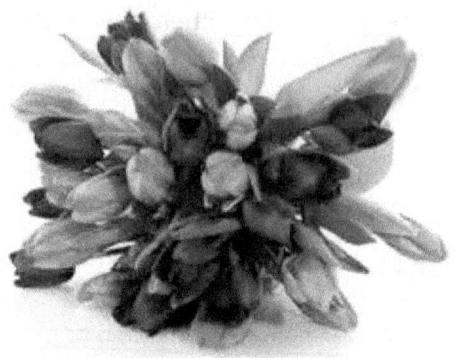

Special Thanks

I would like to offer my sincere and heartfelt thanks to St Vincent Carmel Hospital, St. Vincent Bariatric Weight Loss Center of Excellence, Dr. Margaret Inman and all the dieticians, nurses and hospital staff for assisting me in my weight loss journey. My personal physician, Dr. Chris LaFollette was also an encouraging factor in my weight loss efforts.

I would also like to thank my husband, Rick Frazier and my son, Ryan Frazier for offering me support and encouragement when I needed it the most.

---Sophia Frazier

My Personal Journey Through Bariatric Surgery

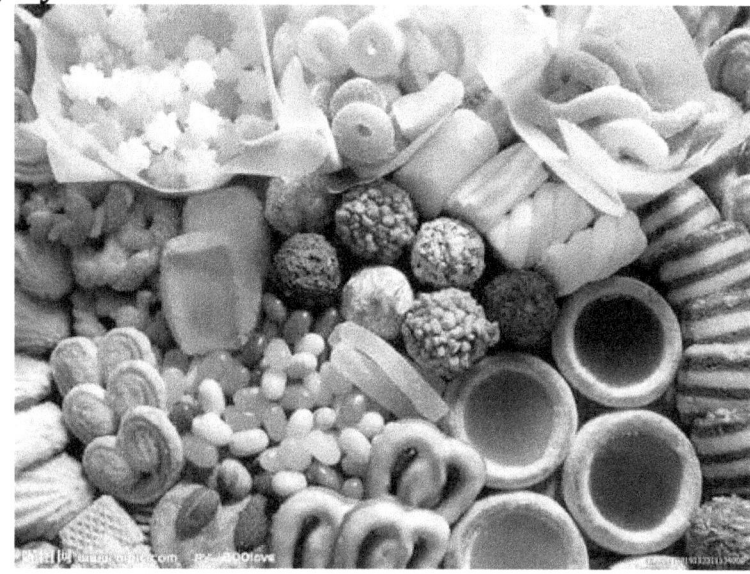

My Childhood

I've always been prone to weight gain even as a child. I was what I like to call a "yo-yo." I would go through stages where I would slim down some but I was always a "little chubby."

I was not an active child, but preferred the solitary activities such as reading, writing, watching TV etc. Even though I was encouraged, I had no interest in playing team sports and considered myself to be quite awkward. I was usually one of the last ones chosen for a team so why would I subject myself to the humiliation?

Only those who have dealt with it understand the humiliation of being called fat. It is very hurtful and tends to cause the individual to isolate themselves all the more so that they don't have to deal with the pain of rejection.

My mother was constantly trying to limit my access to food and telling me that I needed to lose weight. I know that

My Personal Journey Through Bariatric Surgery

she had good intentions, but all that her efforts did was cause me to hoard food in my room and binge in private.

I used food as a comfort. If I had a bad day I would soothe myself by treating myself with a favorite food. It could be anything from chicken soup to a Twinkie. It would just depend on my mood at the time. It also would not be unusual for me to eat a whole box of Twinkies in one day if I needed a lot of comforting.

Food would make me feel better while I ate it, but then after I ate it I would feel guilty about it. By feeling guilty, I needed more comfort, hence more food. It became a vicious cycle that became more pronounced as I got older.

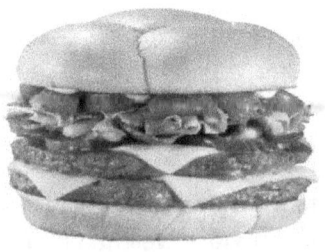

My Personal Journey Through Bariatric Surgery

My Addiction to Food

As an adult, through many trials and tribulations I discovered that I was addicted to food. Some people want cigarettes, drugs or alcohol but my pleasure was food. People don't understand that it is actually easier to quit cigarettes, drugs or alcohol than it is to stop an addiction to food. A person can abstain from the other addictions, but a person needs to eat regardless of an addiction. I'm not saying that other addictions are easy to overcome, for they are definitely not, but food is a requirement for life.

Some people will tell you to just stop eating and push the plate away. This is easier said by a skinny person who is not addicted to the pleasures of eating.

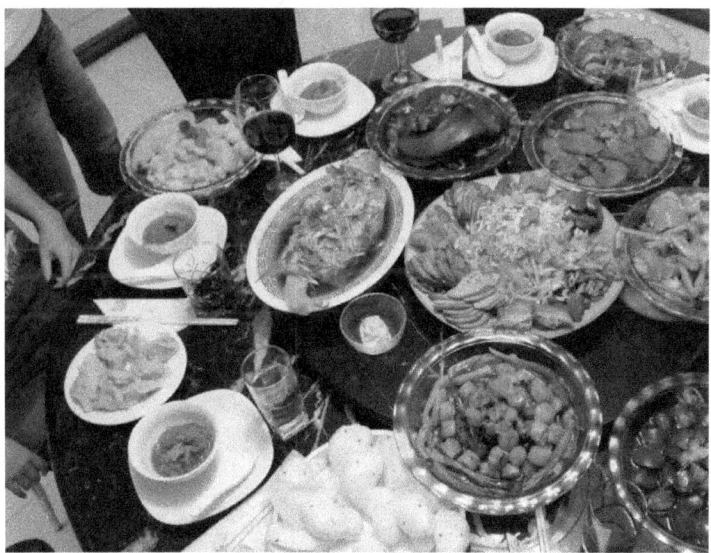

I have at times fasted for weight loss and it gave me a sense of power and control when I lost weight. I just didn't realize at the time that I was actually making my overall weight problem worse. The body is very efficient at conserving calories when it thinks it is starving. This means that when I did it, my body was more likely to store the calories as fat for my next "starvation."

My Personal Journey Through Bariatric Surgery

Weight would become harder and harder to lose.

Most social activities that people participate in are centered on food in some way. Family get gatherings are usually over a large pot luck meal. People go out for dinner or go to the movies and eat popcorn. The list just goes on. A social gathering is usually centered on the presentation and consumption of food in some form.

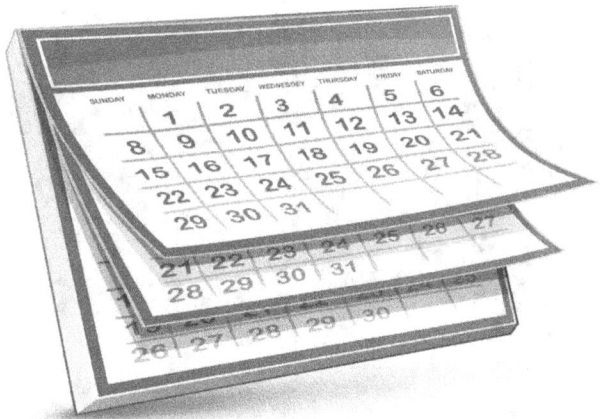

The Past

I have always had a poor body image of myself. Even when I was thin, I didn't feel thin. I was my own worst critic. I didn't feel comfortable in social settings because I was worried about my appearance.

I got to a point where I thought what was the use in trying? I just knew that I would fail at maintaining my weight anyway. This truly led to my downfall. I would eat more to

My Personal Journey Through Bariatric Surgery

comfort myself. I would then resort to buying larger clothes to hide the fact I was gaining weight or so I thought. I then began avoiding social situations because I didn't want anyone to see how much weight that I had gained. I was miserable and ashamed of myself. Eventually something had to give.

In 2000, I underwent a procedure that was called a "stomach staple" in layman's terms for weight loss. It worked for a time. I actually lost over 100 lbs. and felt wonderful. After a few years, I learned that it's a good idea to make sure that your surgeon is board certified for bariatric surgery. Many people do not realize that any surgeon can perform the surgery, but it does not mean that they are specifically trained to perform bariatric procedures.

A board certified bariatric surgeon is required to undergo a specific amount of study and prove that they can understand and perform the standard procedures. Until the surgeon is tested and approved for certification then he or she does not have the required training. This lack of training can result in badly performed procedures and lifelong medical issues for the recipient of the surgical procedure.

I began having problems with acid reflux and severe heartburn. I also began gaining my weight back. To determine what the exact nature of the problem was I underwent several tests including an endoscopy to learn the nature of my problems. The physician who performed the procedure informed me that I had an untreated hiatal hernia, esophagitis and my prior surgery was coming undone and causing some of my symptoms.

The physician who performed the endoscopy also told me that I only had a couple of options to alleviate my symptoms. One was to consider taking a drug that was not approved by the FDA for use in the United States and risking developing tardive dyskinesia or having surgical repair of the hernia and a revision of my prior bariatric surgery.

My Personal Journey Through Bariatric Surgery

At first I did try taking the drug that he gave as an option. This meant I would have to order it from a pharmacy outside of the United States. One of the reasons that it was not approved by the FDA was that drug companies in the U.S. could not find a reason to get it approved. There was no profit in it and they could not recoup the start up cost of getting it approved.

I eventually opted to try the surgical revision because the medication was difficult for me to obtain and the risk of side effects worried me. I also determined that the medication did little to alleviate my symptoms.

The surgical option requires research to find qualified surgeons and determining the best facilities for the surgical procedure. I investigated several facilities and learned that my prior surgery and complications limited me as to where I could go. I definitely needed a physician who was highly qualified to perform the surgery and a facility that could provide the care that I would need if there were any complications. Is the surgical option dangerous? No more so than any other surgery when put under anesthetics. There are risks inherent with any medical procedure.

My Personal Journey Through Bariatric Surgery

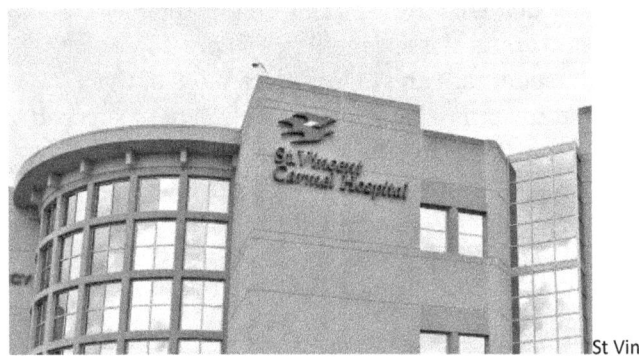
St Vincent Hospital in Carmel, Indiana

My Choice

I chose the Bariatric Center at St. Vincent Carmel Hospital located at 13500 North Meridian Street in Carmel, Indiana. It wasn't the closest to me, but it met the criteria that I required. They had a highly experienced medical staff who dealt specifically with bariatric patients. Another plus was that quite a few employees there had undergone bariatric surgery themselves so they were well aware of what a potential patient would need to undergo to be successful. It also made it easier for me to ask questions as many of those professionals that I asked had actually experienced the procedure.

As a potential patient prior to being accepted into their program, I had to take an educational seminar. The free seminar was an introduction to the procedures available and qualifications that must be met before a client can be approved for the procedure.

Even though I had a bariatric procedure previously with all the medical advances I needed to be informed of my choices.

My Personal Journey Through Bariatric Surgery

To be a bariatric patient at St. Vincent it is the policy that seminar attendance is required. I think meeting others who were experiencing making the same choices made it easier to make such an important decision in my life.

This particular facility offers counseling, support groups, cooking classes, exercise classes, medical and pre-surgery consultations, hospital care and follow up care. All of this support is geared toward helping the bariatric patient succeed in weight loss and maintenance.

Family members are encouraged to support the potential patient and participate in the decision making process. The candidates who are most successful have the support of others in their daily lives.

They also offer assistance with getting insurance approval for the procedure and getting medical leave or FMLA paperwork properly filled out for the patient's employer.

My Personal Journey Through Bariatric Surgery

The Requirements

To be accepted as a potential bariatric surgery patient requires an individual to be considered morbidly obese. To obtain the diagnosis of morbid obesity an individual is diagnosed using the *Body Mass Index* or BMI.

BMI is determined by using a ration of height to weight. Normal BMI readings are between 20-25 and those who are morbidly obese have readings over 40 and tend to be at least 100 lbs. over their ideal body weight. Individuals with a BMI of 35 or less are usually encouraged to use nonsurgical means for weight loss. My reading was over 40.

Those who are dealing with obesity tend to be more susceptible to health conditions such as high blood pressure, diabetes, sleep apnea, heart disease, osteoarthritis, cancer, gall stones and gastroesophageal reflux also known as GERD (Highland Hospital Bariatric Center 2012).

I happen to be one of those who are susceptible. I have high blood pressure, osteoarthritis, GERD, esophagitis and low thyroid function. I take on average seven prescription medications per day to combat medical issues that have not been resolved.

There can be multiple reasons for being overweight. It can be due to heredity, a medical condition, overeating or a combination of things. Many people who are overweight don't feel well and find it difficult to complete activities that can lead to weight loss and better health. Individuals who are of average weight may not understand the problems inherent with extra pounds.

My Personal Journey Through Bariatric Surgery

Adult BMI Chart

BMI	19	20	21	22	23	24	25	26	27	28	29	30	31	32	33	34	35
Height							Weight in Pounds										
4'10"	91	96	100	105	110	115	119	124	129	134	138	143	148	153	158	162	167
4'11"	94	99	104	109	114	119	124	128	133	138	143	148	153	158	163	168	173
5'	97	102	107	112	118	123	128	133	138	143	148	153	158	163	168	174	179
5'1"	100	106	111	116	122	127	132	137	143	148	153	158	164	169	174	180	185
5'2"	104	409	115	120	126	131	136	142	147	153	158	164	169	175	180	186	191
5'3"	107	113	118	124	130	135	141	146	152	158	163	169	175	180	186	191	197
5'4"	110	116	122	128	134	140	145	151	157	163	169	174	180	186	192	197	204
5'5"	114	120	123	132	138	144	150	156	162	168	174	180	186	192	198	204	210
5'6"	118	124	130	136	142	148	155	161	167	173	179	186	192	198	204	210	216
5'7"	121	127	134	140	146	153	159	166	172	178	185	191	198	204	211	217	223
5'8"	125	131	138	144	151	158	164	171	177	184	190	197	203	210	216	223	230
5'9"	128	135	142	149	155	162	169	176	182	189	196	203	209	216	223	230	236
5'10"	132	139	146	153	160	167	174	181	188	195	202	209	216	222	229	236	243
5'11"	136	143	150	157	165	172	179	186	193	200	208	215	222	229	236	243	250
6'	140	147	154	162	169	177	184	191	199	206	213	221	228	235	242	250	258
6'1"	144	151	159	166	174	182	189	197	204	212	219	227	235	242	250	257	265
6'2"	148	155	163	171	179	186	194	202	210	218	225	233	241	249	256	264	272
6'3"	152	160	168	176	184	192	200	208	216	224	232	240	248	256	264	272	279
	Healthy Weight						Overweight					Obese					

BMI Chart

My Personal Journey Through Bariatric Surgery

Surgical Options

There are three types of surgical options which include restrictive, malabsorptive and a combination of the other two. Restrictive procedures make the stomach smaller to decrease food intake while malabsorptive lessens the amount of intestine that comes in contact with the food. This prevents the body from absorbing as many calories from the food.

These procedures can be performed in one of two ways. The first is through an open incision which can be between 4-7 inches in length on the abdomen. The recuperation time for this surgery is on average 6-8 weeks.

The second option is laparascopic. The recovery time for this surgical procedure is anywhere from 2-4 weeks. This surgery is performed by creating several smaller incisions in the abdomen to accommodate a small video camera and the instruments themselves (St Vincent Carmel Hospital, 2013).

Depending on prior surgeries and other unforeseen circumstances an open incision may be necessary for an individual. The laparoscopic procedure is generally more desired as the risk of infection and recovery time is much less.

My Personal Journey Through Bariatric Surgery

Expected Weight Loss

<u>One to Three Months Post-Surgery</u>-Weight loss will depend on how well an individual is following the physicians recommendations.

<u>Six Months After Surgery</u>-with gastric bypass surgery, a loss of 30% to 40% of excess body weight is entirely possible.

☐   <u>Nine Months Post-Surgery-Vitamin</u> deficiencies or lack of sufficient weight loss are noticeable at this time.

☐   <u>One Year After Surgery</u>-Between 12 to 18 months after surgery a 100 lb weight loss isn't unusual.

Keep in mind the excess weight did not appear overnight and it will take more than overnight to lose it.

My Personal Journey Through Bariatric Surgery

Surgical Types

The types of surgery available are dependent upon the facility that is chosen and the expertise of the surgeons themselves. Possible surgery types include Adjustable Gastric Banding, Sleeve Gastrectomy, Biliopancreatic Diversion, Roux-n-Y and others. Each type of surgery has its positive and negative aspects and it is a very good idea to research what may be best for you under your particular circumstances.

I had researched the options and I had chosen the Gastric Sleeve. Upon meeting with my physician, Dr. Margaret Inman and her reviewing my medical past she informed me that the Gastric Sleeve would not be an option due to my prior surgery and the scarring inherent with it. She suggested a Roux-n-Y as it would be more successful for me and have the least risk.

After some thought, I decided that it would be best to accept the medical advice she had given me. I agreed to the Roux-n-Y procedure. The Roux-n-Y procedure can be associated with frequent diarrhea (also known as dumping syndrome) and failure to absorb enough calcium and iron.

There are risks with any medical procedure and medical personnel are required to provide a potential patient with possible risks inherent with a specific surgical procedure. Those risks are possibilities not probabilities. It doesn't necessarily mean that an individual will have that problem after surgery.

My Personal Journey Through Bariatric Surgery

Possible Future Procedures

I needed to keep in mind the possibility for future surgical procedures. Some individuals who undergo weight loss surgery may find unwanted physical side effects especially if the weight loss is dramatic. Losing a large amount of weight can lead to excessive skin flab. Exercise may help tone the body but might not be able to rid it of a large amount of excessive skin. I also need to realize that insurance may balk at performing procedures that it considers to be cosmetic such as: a lower body lift, thigh lift, arm lift, breast lift or a tummy tuck. Each person is unique and not everyone would need additional procedures or want them. The elasticity of the skin is different for everyone. Nutrition, genetics, amount of weight loss, age of the person and multiple other factors play a part. Will I consider other procedures for myself? Honestly, I don't know at this point. I just want to lose weight.

My Personal Journey Through Bariatric Surgery

Physicians

At the Carmel Center there are several physicians who are highly qualified in different types of bariatric surgery and weight loss techniques. I felt quite comfortable knowing that I would receive quality care which was of importance to me. My physician:

Margaret Inman M.D., F.A.C.S.A Chicago native, Dr. Inman is a graduate of the University of Illinois-Chicago, with a master's degree in biology, and also of Indiana University School of Medicine. Dr. Inman completed her general surgery residency at Methodist Hospital of Indiana. She is a fellow of the American College of Surgeons, board-certified by the American Board of Surgery and a member of the American Society for Bariatric Surgery. Dr. Inman has performed bariatric surgery since 1997, and she specializes in bariatric laparoscopic procedures including the Gastric Band, Roux-en-y and duodenal switch (St. Vincent).

My Personal Journey Through Bariatric Surgery

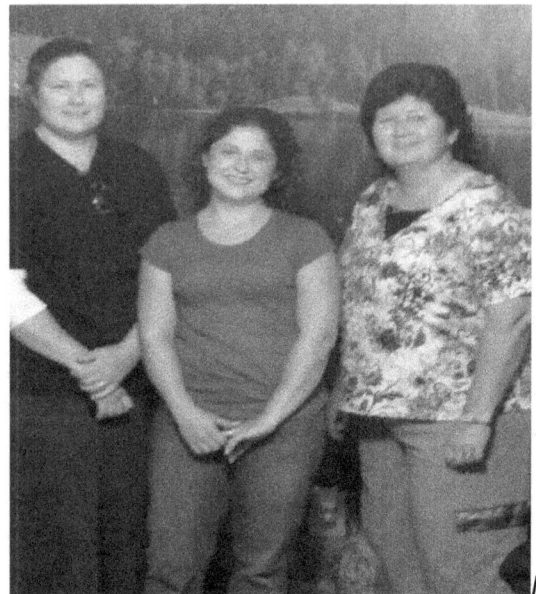

Illustration 1:

BEFORE SURGERY: ME ON THE RIGHT

Time Line

<u>February 2012</u>   I attended required informational seminar to become a bariatric patient at St. Vincent. It was free.

I began attending support group once a month for Bariatric patients. Classes were in my locality. The classes are free and I made new friends who were able to share their experiences and give advice. They are chaired by a trained individual such as a nurse or someone who has undergone the procedure themselves.

I notified my primary care physician of my tentative plans. He tries to aid my weight loss through the use of diet and exercise. He keeps detailed records for me in case the insurance requires me to try other alternatives first.

My Personal Journey Through Bariatric Surgery

<u>March 2012</u> My primary insurance denies the procedure as they have a clause that says they will not cover anything to do with bariatric procedures regardless of whether or not it is a revision or includes other surgical procedures at the same time. I am so disappointed.

St. Vincent personnel begin the process of checking into my secondary insurance through my husband's employer. My fingers are crossed.

<u>June 2012</u> My work schedule changes so I am no longer able to attend the support group, but I am in contact with the chair by email. This still gives me answers to my questions when I need it.

<u>November 15, 2012</u> My secondary insurance approves the bariatric procedure! I have a year from that date to get it completed. I am pleased.

One of the downfalls to this approval for me is it's as if I now have a license to eat more since I will be severely limited later. This is not a good thing. I start getting larger portions of the things I like or eating what I know I shouldn't.

<u>December 6, 2012</u> Spent most of day getting required testing done for surgery. I meet with a physician the same day who does a required physical exam to make sure that I can tolerate the surgery.

<u>December 14,</u> 2012 I call St Vincent a week after my tests to see if they have gotten the results yet. They have not. I call the hospital where the tests were run and they fax the results again to make sure St. Vincent has them.

<u>Early January 2013</u> I call St. Vincent wondering why I have not been contacted regarding a surgery date yet. I am transferred to a woman named "Angel." She informs me that Dr. Inman only reviews the records of patients on Mondays and the holidays have her behind. Angel assures me that I can call her to get

My Personal Journey Through Bariatric Surgery

updates as needed.

January 14, 2013 Got surgical date of March 21, 2013 at 9am! Backlog is due to large demand for surgical procedure.

January 15, 2013 Got date of March 7, 2013 to take all day class with dietician from 8:30 am until 4:30 pm. It takes place exactly two weeks before my surgery date.

January 18, 2013 Received paperwork in the mail to fill out for the dietician and my all day class. I review it and plan on filling it out soon. I am getting impatient with waiting.

January 19, 2013 Filled out required paperwork. I was required to list all medications that I take and their dosages on a regular basis. Also, I listed over the counter medications and vitamins. I needed to write down when and where my lab work and physical was done for the surgery.

February, 2013 Waiting…

March 7, 2013 Today I go to my required all day pre-op class. I worked until midnight the night before. I had to get up at 4 am to get ready and be on my way at 5 am. I have at least a 2 hour drive to get to Carmel, IN. I'm already tired and I haven't even started. I'm excited too, because it's starting to become a reality for me.

My class doesn't officially start until 8 am, but they want me there at least an hour to an hour and a half early to fill out paperwork, weigh in and get my "before" picture taken.

At my weigh in, I weigh exactly 247.9 pounds and I am 5' 3 ½" tall. My goal weight would be between 127 pounds and 137 pounds. I'd be happy if I could just lose 40 pounds! I know that I will feel better as long as I lose weight.

I have also been made aware that after surgery, I may not need to continue taking all seven of the prescriptions I now

My Personal Journey Through Bariatric Surgery

take for various medical problems. The weight loss may alleviate some of those problems for me. Even if it does not, I will be healthier for the weight loss.

There are at least 20 to 30 other individuals present for the class. We are all introduced to each other and learn of our surgery dates and surgeons who will be performing the surgeries. Not everyone is having the same surgical procedure, but the care needed after the surgery is very similar.

Many of us will be getting procedures done within days of each other. I will probably see many of our classmates in the hospital at the same time that I am there.

The fact that fellow patients are introduced to each other provides a support system within the hospital setting for us. We can encourage each other as we all know we are trying to lose weight together.

Some people have brought a support person with them to go over all the information that is provided. Since my surgery will be a revision, I am already aware of much of the information that will be given. I choose to attend the class alone.

During the class, I receive an informational booklet. A dietician, a nurse and a successful bariatric candidate are speakers during the class. We also receive spiritual guidance from a Catholic priest who speaks to us and provides a nondenominational prayer for our success.

The booklet is reviewed during class time and questions are answered for those who have them. We are given a list of all of the bariatric dieticians and their contact information so that we can remain well informed about our specific dietary needs after the surgical procedure.

We are then given specific guidelines as to our diet on the day prior to our surgeries. I am given instructions to eat a

My Personal Journey Through Bariatric Surgery

light breakfast and a full liquid lunch. My dinner is to be clear liquids only and nothing to eat or drink after midnight.

A list of examples of food that will fulfill the requirements is given. Each of us is also instructed regarding how to take medications the morning of surgery or to withhold them. It will vary from person to person dependent upon their specific health needs.

My Personal Journey Through Bariatric Surgery

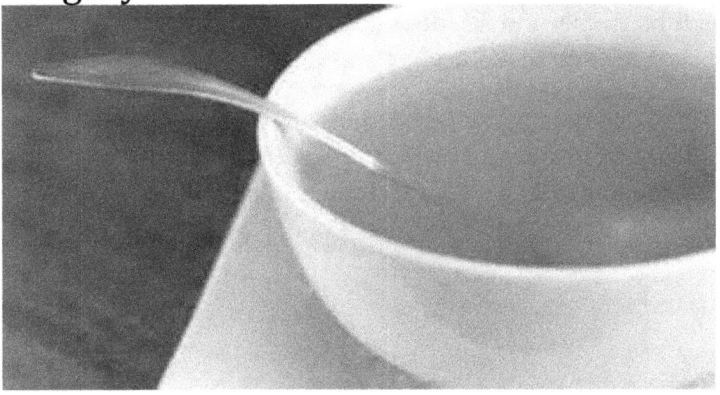

HOSPITAL DIET

The dietician tells us that after surgery we will have specific food intake requirements. On the day of the surgery, I can only have ice chips. This will give my surgery site some rest before I try to consume foods in my vastly changed digestive system.

On the day after surgery, if my system will tolerate it, then I may advance to a clear liquid diet. The items that I can have are very specific and given in small amounts of one to two ounces at a time. These items will also be offered at specific intervals throughout the day.

The second day after surgery, I may be offered full liquid foods. Again, these are very specific items and I can only advance to this next stage of foods after I have tolerated the previous stage. The easiest way to determine if I can tolerate the foods is if my body will allow me to keep the food down. If I were to vomit or have other gastrointestinal distress then I am not ready for the next stage. It will take time and it varies with the individual.

An individual's surgeon may change the diet plan at any time for a specific patient. This may be due to the patient's unique needs. Also, just because patient A can tolerate clear

My Personal Journey Through Bariatric Surgery

liquids on the second day does not mean that patients B or C can advance to that stage yet and so on.

According to the Mayo Clinic, dehydration is a possible complication following a weight loss procedure. An individual is no longer able to drink large quantities of liquid at one time.

My Personal Journey Through Bariatric Surgery

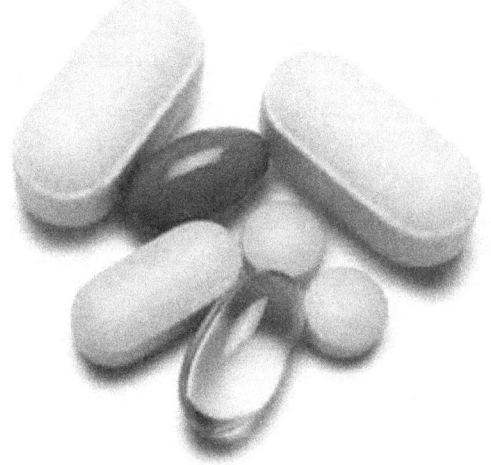

LIFELONG VITAMIN SUPPLEMENTS REQUIRED

The dietician explains that due to a drastic change in my digestive system, I will need to supplement my food intake with a variety of vitamins to prevent malnutrition. After weight loss surgical procedures, my body may not absorb certain vitamins and minerals that it needs. I will be required to take multivitamins, iron, calcium citrate, vitamin D3, Thiamine, and B12. A probiotic is also recommended but not required. My physician through regular lab work will determine my specific requirements.

These supplements are to be taken in specific amounts along with a strict diet regimen to meet all the daily nutritional requirements. Instruction is also provided on what brands of supplements meet the requirements needed. Not all brands provide the specific nutritional needs of a bariatric patient.

Also, I need to realize that I may need to space out my intake of vitamin supplements and prescription medicines throughout the day rather than trying to ingest them all at once.

My Personal Journey Through Bariatric Surgery

My stomach may not tolerate a large quantity of pills.

According to the Mayo Clinic weight-reduction surgery may result in:

Anemia due to deficiency of iron or vitamin B12
Neurologic complications from vitamin B12 deficiency
Kidney stone disease due to changes in how the body absorbs calcium and oxalate
Possible bone disease due to mineral or vitamin D deficiency

My Personal Journey Through Bariatric Surgery

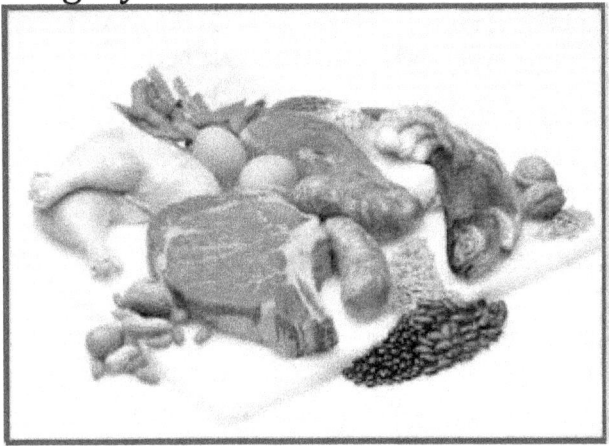

SPECIFIC PROTEIN REQUIREMENTS

The body needs a significant amount of protein to function normally. A bariatric patient's diet is so restricted that the individual must prioritize ingestion of protein to prevent a disease. The disease is known as Protein Calorie Malnutrition (PCM).

PCM can lead to hair loss, muscle loss, a lack of energy and poor healing. Protein is needed to maintain the function of body organs and skeletal muscles.

I learn that five days after surgery, I will need to begin ingesting protein supplements just to meet my body's requirements. I can start the supplements only if my body has tolerated the diet changes so far. If it has not, I may need to wait before starting the protein supplements. I know that since my stomach will be about the size of a walnut that I cannot obtain all the protein I need for a day's nutrition without supplementing my diet somehow.

The dietician provides a list of the amount of protein a human body needs and specific protein supplement options that meet the requirements. It is stressed that there are other

My Personal Journey Through Bariatric Surgery

protein supplement options on the market, but they do not meet the specific needs of the bariatric patient.

According to the Mayo Clinic, in the first three to six months after surgery the body reacts to the rapid loss of weight. Individuals could experience body aches, fatigue, hair loss, mood changes, the inability to regulate temperature changes, dry skin and a condition known as NIPHS.

"Mayo Clinic doctors have recognized and reported on a seemingly rare but serious complication following gastric bypass called non-insulinoma pancreatogenous hypoglycemia syndrome (NIPHS) or post-bariatric surgery hypoglycemia. After a person eats, this condition can result in very low blood sugar levels that lead to severe neurologic symptoms, including visual disturbances, confusion and (rarely) seizures (Mayo Clinic 2013).

My Personal Journey Through Bariatric Surgery

Anatomy of the Abdomen

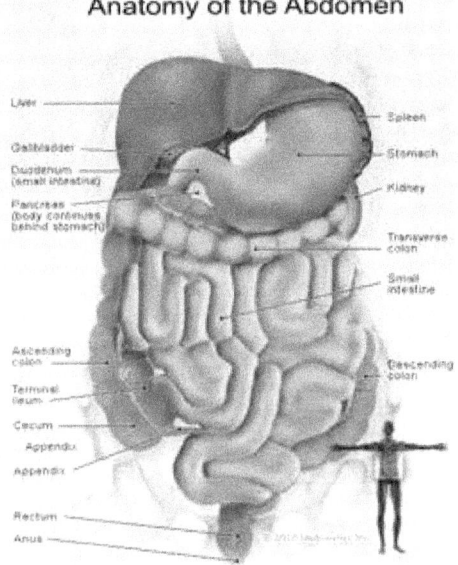

Liver
Gallbladder
Duodenum (small intestine)
Pancreas (body continues behind stomach)
Spleen
Stomach
Kidney
Transverse colon
Small intestine
Ascending colon
Terminal ileum
Cecum
Appendix
Appendix
Descending colon
Rectum
Anus

DUMPING SYNDROME

Dumping syndrome may occur because a large portion of the stomach and intestine has been bypassed because of bariatric surgery. The symptoms of the syndrome may include feelings of weakness, sweating, nausea, dizziness, rapid heartbeat, lowered blood pressure, cramping and diarrhea.

My Personal Journey Through Bariatric Surgery

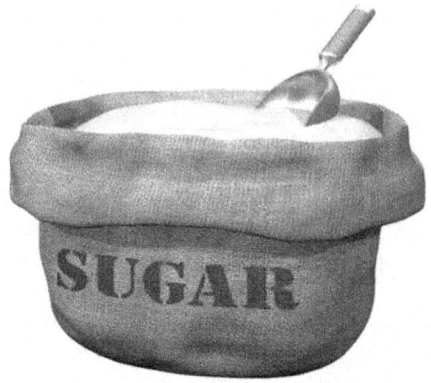

The easiest method to avoid dumping syndrome is to restrict sugar and fat intake. The redesigned digestive system is not able to endure the same amount of sugar and fat intake prior to surgery.

I've also been informed by the dietician that my own personal tastes are likely to change because of the surgery. I may not want as much sugar or fat in my diet. I think that this is a good thing!

HYPOGLYCEMIA

Hypoglycemia can occur in individuals who have had bariatric surgery. The condition of low blood sugar can happen to a patient even if there is no prior history of diabetes. Symptoms may include: faintness, dizziness, hunger, blurred vision, trembling, anxiety and irritability.

Low blood sugar is caused primarily during a rapid delivery of food into the small intestine. The food may cause excess production of insulin secretion which in turn may lead to lower blood sugar levels.

Recommendations to avoid hypoglycemia include not going over three hours without eating. Eat small mixed meals and snacks that include complex carbohydrates, proteins and fiber. Avoid alcohol, caffeine and simple sugars.

My Personal Journey Through Bariatric Surgery

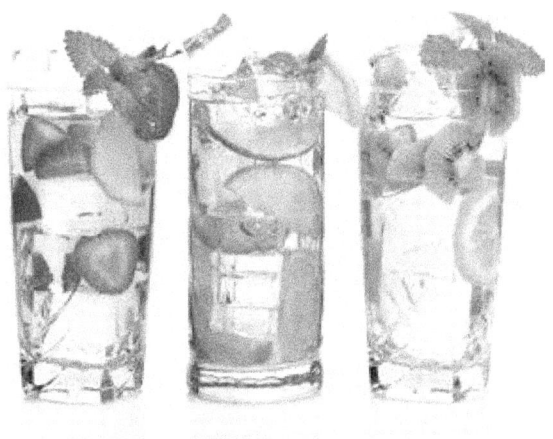

DEHYDRATION

After surgery dehydration can occur since the patient does not have the stomach capacity to hold a large amount of liquid. The symptoms of dehydration can include: nausea, fatigue, body aches, headache, lightheadedness and dry mouth.

Remember to sip fluids throughout the day between meals. Try to drink at least 64 ounces of fluid daily. Enlist different flavorings to enhance the taste of the drink.

My Personal Journey Through Bariatric Surgery

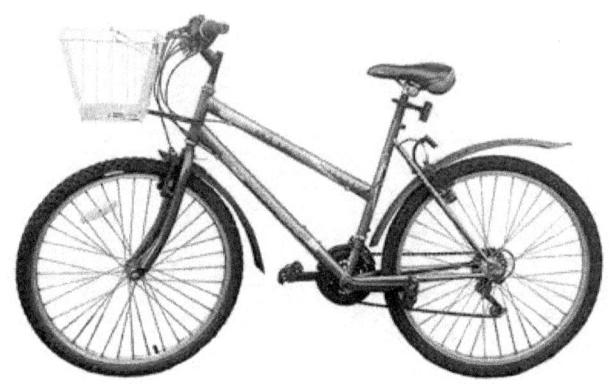

LIFE STYLE CHANGES

A bariatric patient must make permanent life style changes to be successful in weight loss and maintaining health. Several changes include eating three meals a day, eating slowly, and drink at least 64-80 ounces of low calorie fluids daily.

Avoiding alcoholic, caffeinated and carbonated beverages is highly recommended. These beverages can contain empty calories, increase digestive discomfort and cause "dumping syndrome."

Physical activity of at least five hours per week is also recommended for maximum weight loss and regulation of the body's systems.

A daily journal should be kept to log nutritional intake and activity levels. It's much easier to monitor what requirements have been met by reviewing a written record of it.

My Personal Journey Through Bariatric Surgery

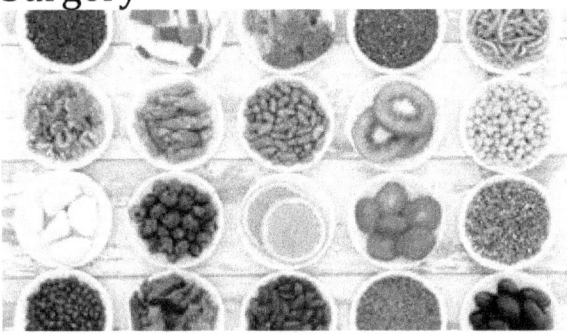

MEAL PLANS

During class, I am provided with a general guideline as to what can be expected after surgery. The exact diet an individual follows must be determined by the physician. The meal plans are developed to promote rapid weight loss, to maintain weight loss, to promote health and prevent any adverse side effects from the procedure.

For the weeks following the surgery a patient make expect different stages in the diet. For the first month after surgery, a completely liquid diet is the norm. Specific dietary items are provided on a list to aid in recovery from surgery and provide nutritional needs. It is stressed that if an item is not listed on your dietary plan then DO NOT EAT IT. The chances are you will experience extreme discomfort and possible vomiting by not following instructions!

At 5 to 8 weeks after surgery, the patient may move on to pureed foods as tolerated. These items must come from the provided list of choices.

From 9 to 15 weeks, a bariatric patient may expect to move past pureed foods as tolerated. Again, there is a list provided of specific choices. Do not stray from the list.

At 4 months to 6 months the volume of food may increase. At 7 months to 9 months the volume of food may

My Personal Journey Through Bariatric Surgery

increase again as tolerated. There are stage changes at months 10 to 12, 12 to 18 months and beyond 18 months. These changes may include increased volume and food choices.

These stages may vary somewhat due to your specific requirements and the recommendations of the physician and dietician. FOLLOW THE PLAN AS DIRECTED.

While at the all-day class I bought supplements at the women's boutique in the hospital during lunch hour. These items will be replacements for what I cannot eat.

I also stopped in Dr. Inman's office to make sure that my paperwork was up to date for my leave of absence from work.

March 8, 2013 I bought liquid food items and stored them for future use. I contacted my pharmacy to inquire about getting more digestible medications if physician continues them after my hospital release.

March 9, 2013 I caught up on chores and paperwork. I went ahead and packed a bag for my hospital stay. I also talked to my husband about what to expect and what needed to be arranged. I had a conversation with my adult son about upcoming procedure. What I did was reviewed everything with both of them for myself as well as them.

March 10, 2013 Today I talked to my coworkers about arrangements while I am off of work. Work today was otherwise normal.

March 12, 2013 I'm starting to get nervous and excited. The surgery is little more than a week away. My whole life will change. I wonder how much weight I will lose?

My Personal Journey Through Bariatric Surgery

<u>March 14, 2013</u> I verify with my family physician that my regular prescriptions can be modified to accommodate my needs after surgery. Nurse assures me that they are now called in to my pharmacy so that they will be ready when I need them.

<u>March 18, 2013</u> I saw the chiropractor today. I haven't been able to take anything stronger than Tylenol since last Thursday in preparation for the surgery. My aches and pains let me know that I had to do something.

<u>March 19, 2013</u> I received a phone call from St. Vincent Bariatric. I am now preregistered for my surgery the day after tomorrow. It's getting real! I did some last minute grocery shopping for myself and my family while I am recuperating. I reviewed my pre-surgery diet for tomorrow. I made sure my bags are ready and set up my prescription medicines for when I come home after the surgery.

<u>March 20, 2013</u> I received a courtesy call from St. Vincent reminding me of my scheduled surgery tomorrow. I am to follow my preop diet (which I am), leave all my jewelry and valuables at home and be THERE at 6:30 am. I work tonight until midnight.

I will have to be up at 3:00 am to shower and get ready. It's at least a 2 hour drive. I am glad my husband is driving! Just maybe I can doze on the way up there. I really doubt that I actually sleep, I'm too anxious!

My diet for today means that I need to eat a light breakfast, a full liquid lunch and only clear liquids for dinner. The hospital has provided me with a list of choices to satisfy the requirements.

My evening at work is hectic taking care of last minute details before going out on leave. I work until 12 am then rush home to lie down for a few short hours of rest.

My Personal Journey Through Bariatric Surgery

<u>March 21, 2013</u> Rick, my husband and I arrive at St. Vincent Carmel Hospital at 5:30 am at the correct entrance for admitting. We are both impressed with the hospital itself and the kindness of the staff. We aren't subject to waiting even though we are an hour early.

There is minimal paperwork left to do at this stage. They merely need to verify my identity through ID and confirm my insurance information. I am taken straight to a reception area for surgical patients while Rick is allowed to have full use of the lounge including complementary coffee and tea until staff are ready to bring him back to my room.

I am definitely nervous, but I am reassured and greeted by nursing staff as they take me to my room where I will prepare and wait for my surgery.

Once I am in my room they again verify my identity and provide me with several arm bands so that hospital staff will have the information regarding my case immediately available as needed. I sign a few consent forms and preparations begin.

A very nice nurse brings in a hospital gown, some pressure hose and some footies for me to wear. I am instructed as to the significance of the hose to prevent blood clots and how to properly wear them. I am given time to change out of my street clothes and into my hospital attire.

The same nurse returns and weighs me one last time before the surgery and gets all my vital signs. I am made comfortable in a hospital bed and given nice heated blankets to stay cozy warm.

At each stage of the process, I am informed as to what will be happening and why and encouraged to ask questions at any time that I need answers. I find this very

My Personal Journey Through Bariatric Surgery

soothing to my somewhat jangled nerves. After all, I don't have surgery every day and this is going to be a life changing event!

The same nurse who greeted me remains throughout the process and introduces me to other members of the staff as needed. My IV is started for fluids as they have found that patients feel better if they remain hydrated while waiting for their procedure. This makes sense to me as I am thirsty from being restricted from taking anything by mouth and have been since midnight. Once the IV is inserted and I am made comfortable, my husband is allowed to come back and sit with me until it's time for the surgery.

While we wait, the surgical nurse, anesthesiologist and surgeon come in to visit us and offer last minute advice as to what to expect and give us an opportunity to ask questions. Time seems to move by very quickly at this stage.

It is finally time for the procedure. I am instructed to walk down to the operating room under my own power and reminded that when I am able after the procedure that I will be walking at two hour intervals to prevent blood clots.

The nurses banter with me about various light subjects while the anesthesiologist explains that once the sedative is placed into my IV that the next thing I know I will be waking up in the recovery room.

When I wake up, I will more than likely be attached to several monitors and possibly two IVs. I will be receiving oxygen through a tube at my nose and I will have a drainage tube and a gastric tube to assist me in my recovery.

True to their word, I remember talking to one of the nurses in the operating room about my adult son. The next thing I remember is waking up in the recovery room attached

My Personal Journey Through Bariatric Surgery

to several monitors. There is some pain, but I am given access to pain medications as I need them. I am very tired.

I am encouraged to breathe deeply and do my best although I am restricted in expanding my abdomen from both the surgery itself and a band placed around my abdomen for support. I recall drifting in and out of a daze for some time before I am fully aware of my surroundings. Rick is with me in the room.

The nurses come in at regular intervals and monitor my vital signs to make sure that they are within normal ranges. I am reminded that as soon as I think I am able that staff will assist me in getting up for a short walk before returning to my bed.

These short walks will occur on an average of every two hours for at least twenty four hours following surgery. They are used as a preventative to blood clots and pneumonia. Being overweight puts added stress on the chest cavity and lungs, resulting in a greater risk of pneumonia after the surgery. The walking assists the body in processing the medications left in the body from the surgical procedure. The more often I am able to move about the sooner the medications will dissipate.

I gather my courage and agree to a short walk around the bariatric floor. For the first walk, I am very unsteady on my feet and use the IV pole to brace myself on while I am trailed by my husband and two nursing staff to make sure that I do not fall. I return to my room completely drained of strength and with assistance I am put to bed. I fall into a restless sleep until the next round of walking.

My routine for the next twenty four hours consists of nothing but walking, sleeping and ingesting ice chips for thirst. I am on IV fluids to prevent any need for anything

My Personal Journey Through Bariatric Surgery

else. This allows my digestive system time to heal.

I gradually begin to notice other patients on my floor following the same routine that I am. The center handles a significant number of bariatric patients daily. I also begin to notice that some are more motivated than others. Usually the ones with family support present seem more motivated. Family is an encouraging factor.

March 22, 2013 I remain in the hospital and my husband is provided with a recliner so that he may stay in my room with me. My adult son is holding down the fort at home. It is a great comfort knowing that everything is being taken care of while I am unable to do it myself.

I continue the walking routine. Rick assists me in taking a shower and washing my hair. I feel so much more human once this is done!

I am offered the option of clear liquids by mouth, but I continue to prefer the ice chips. I still sleep much of the time.

March 23 and March 24, 2013 I remain in the hospital improving daily. During this time I progress to eating small amounts of pureed foods. The drainage tube and IVs are removed. I am given the option of being released to go home providing I follow their strict guidelines. I readily agree.

That evening, I rest in a recliner in my own home. It is still too difficult to get in and out of my own bed so the recliner becomes my friend for a few days.

March 26, 2013 I am starting to get into a routine at home and appear to have more energy and feel better each day. I must remain in the habit of walking to increase blood flow

My Personal Journey Through Bariatric Surgery

and prevent blood clots.

On a daily basis, I sleep until I wake on my own, take my medications as directed and watch my dietary intake. I really have no desire for anything, but I follow doctor's orders. I do take prescription medication for pain as I am still extremely sore and my abdominal muscles protest loudly when I move about too much. That's to be expected with the type of surgery I endured.

March 29, 2013   Today is the first day that I have opted to dress after taking a shower rather than return to a clean robe and gown. I'm wearing a T-shirt and sweatpants to prevent discomfort due to constriction or chafing. I still plan on remaining at home and recuperating. My house dog sure seems to enjoy my company on a daily basis at this point. When I am able to go back to work, the dog will probably miss my company.

NOTE TO SELF: Drink more fluids to prevent dehydration. It is easy to tell when I am not ingesting enough fluids as urine becomes more concentrated and has a stronger odor.

April 1, 2013 I've slept in my own bed the past two nights instead of the recliner. I'm much more comfortable and I am using pain medication intermittently rather than daily now. I was able to clean my house and cook a meal for my family without discomfort.

April 2, 2013 I have been taking shots daily of blood thinner since my return home from the hospital. This is an added precaution to prevent blood clots because of the surgery and my reduced activity level. Tonight, I took the last needed shot!

I never have been a fan of needles and I think that I

My Personal Journey Through Bariatric Surgery

dreaded the self-administration of the shots worse than the actual surgical procedure, *but* I've found that it wasn't nearly as bad as I thought it would be. The end results have kept me motivated and it helped when I had a devoted husband who was willing to give me the injections at times.

April 3, 2013   NOTE TO SELF: Try to keep an accurate journal of all food and liquid intake and physical activity no matter how trivial. It all counts toward the final goal of weight loss.

April 6, 2013 I did some laundry today. I also plan on doing some grocery shopping later. My husband has agreed to go with me to do the lifting and carrying. I still get occasional twinges of pain in my abdominal area if I bend certain ways or move too swiftly.

   Some people might be able to go back to work at this point. It's been over two weeks since my surgical procedure. I personally prefer to remain at home a little while longer to recuperate.

April 8, 2013   I'm spending more and more time walking about outdoors. The weather has started to cooperate and my dog is ecstatic with all the walks!

        Both my husband and I have noticed that the swelling in my stomach has gone down quite a bit. I also think that my face appears slightly thinner to me, but that may just be wishful thinking. We'll find out what the doctor thinks on my first visit since the surgery on April 15, 2013.

April 15, 2013 Today I make the trip to Carmel, IN to visit my dietician and my surgeon post-op. According to the dietician, I have lost 21 lbs since my surgery date of March 21, 2013! Yay! I hadn't been weighing myself, but had been concentrating on getting well.

        I felt that it was better not to weigh myself daily as

My Personal Journey Through Bariatric Surgery

weight does fluctuate because of many factors. Also, if I weigh myself only once a week or less then I will be more encouraged by the more dramatic changes in my weight over time.

Since everyone is different, individuals need to be aware that the rapidity of weight loss is dependent on many factors. One's age, sex and health as well as the amount of extra weight an individual is carrying can create different results. The willingness to follow the given dietary and exercise guidelines also plays an important part. No one should be discouraged as long as there is progress.

The dietician after talking to me recommended that I advance to the next stage of my diet, which included pureed foods. I myself prefer to use a food processor or mash the foods to the desired consistency rather than try to eat baby food.

She also recommended that I make sure that I am ingesting at least 75-90 grams of protein per day. I believe that I can do that as well.

When I spoke to Dr. Margaret Inman she said that I was doing well and that she didn't need to see me for three months. I asked about having my gastric tube removed and she had me schedule an appointment for the following week to have it taken out in the office. The procedure was very simple, but she needed to wait until my internal incisions had healed well enough before removing it. I am glad that I no longer needed it!

The gastric tube is placed as a precaution if someone is unable to eat or drink the necessary amounts and becomes dehydrated. I wasn't having a problem with this so it could be removed.

May 1, 2013 I noticed I began to have some abdominal pain and thought that it might be a kidney or bladder infection. I continued my normal routine.

My Personal Journey Through Bariatric Surgery

May 2, 2013 The pain has worsened so I decide to go to the local medical clinic. I did find out that I have lost 33 lbs! I also have a kidney and bladder infection.

Later in the day I feel worse and worse. I end up in the local hospital emergency room. They determine not only do I have a kidney and bladder infection, but I also have a perforated ulcer. I am sent to Carmel Bariatric Center and admitted for treatment and testing. I spend a couple of days in the hospital.

May 3, 2013 Remain hospitalized.

May 4,2013 I am sent home with specific instructions to return for an endoscopy in 6-8 weeks. Due to my bariatric surgery, I am more susceptible to ulcers. An ulcer is an uncommon complication that can develop. The condition is more likely to develop in someone who takes aspirin or other non-steroidal anti-inflammatory agents. I must take medication daily for acid reduction and coating the lining of my stomach.

May 5, 2013 I have reevaluated my diet and have eliminated foods that are spicy, greasy or acidic as they can create problems for someone who is susceptible to ulcers.

May 15, 2013 Last night while preparing to sleep, I was tossing around and inadvertently crossed my legs at the knee for a time. It then dawned on me, I had lost enough weight that I could actually cross my legs at the knee! I went to sleep actually feeling thinner. I knew I wasn't thin, but the possibility that I could be was a pleasant thought! My world had just expanded, while my weight had decreased!

May 30, 2013 I weighed in at the doctor's office today. I have lost a total of 42 lbs., so far! Simply amazing!

July 2013 I no longer take medication for my stomach for ulcers. For me, it is no longer necessary. The doctor agreed. I pay closer attention to what I eat. I watch the types of food, the

My Personal Journey Through Bariatric Surgery

amount of spices and the portions more regularly.

<u>August 2013</u> I will actually get into a bathing suit now. I like being able to relax in the pool and not feel so self conscious. I didn't like the idea of looking like a beached whale or at least feeling as if I looked like one.

<u>October 2013</u> I'm horseback riding again! I can actually mount the horse with no assistance again. I also don't feel sorry for the horse by packing my weight around.

<u>November/December 2013</u> Putting on weight around the holidays had always been a concern for me. I didn't gain anything this time around! I was so proud of myself!

<u>February 2014</u> I like to shop for new clothes again! I am actually enjoying putting outfits together that are stylish and in smaller sizes.

<u>March 2014</u> It's been a year since my weight loss surgery. I have a whole new life. I've lost 100 lbs since the surgery. Could I lose more? Yes, I could probably lose another 20 lbs and be just fine. I am happy where I am weight wise. I never planned on being skinny, I just wanted to lose enough weight that I could be active again.

I exercise at the gym five days a week on a regular basis now. My weight has stabilized. Now it is time to maintain the number that I see on the scales.

<u>February 2014</u>

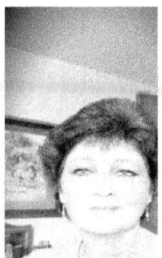

My Personal Journey Through Bariatric Surgery

<u>March 2014</u> I started a new job this month that I never would have attempted before. Success in one area of my life encouraged me to attempt new things in other areas of my life.

<u>April 2014- November 2014</u> Wow! I haven't written anything because I have been too busy out living my life! Training for my new job, horseback riding, motorcycle riding, swimming, camping, etc. I still exercise five days a week. I eat regular meals and snacks but I now automatically consider nutritional content and portion size without thinking about it.

New hair style! Changing the way I wear my make up!

<u>December 2014</u> I still try to work out at least five times a week. I miss it when I don't!

I weigh 136 lbs and I wear a size 8. I actually like shopping for clothes for myself! I can go out to dinner with my friends and eat a small meal. I am satisfied with much less food than before my surgery. I will admit that when I start to overeat I begin getting uncomfortable so my own body tells me when I must stop even if my mind doesn't.

<u>January 2015</u> I weigh 132 lbs now. I don't plan on losing any more weight. I continue to exercise four to five days per week. It doesn't have to be in the gym as keeping it varied makes me more likely to continue to exercise.

I am still glad that I had the surgery done. It has changed my life for the better. I actually feel like living again. Does the surgical procedure mean I can't gain the weight back? No. It simply makes it more difficult for me to consume a large amount of calories.

Remember the journey to weight loss is your personal journey. No one else can do it for you. Only YOU can make it a success story.

My Personal Journey Through Bariatric Surgery

peterkfitness.com

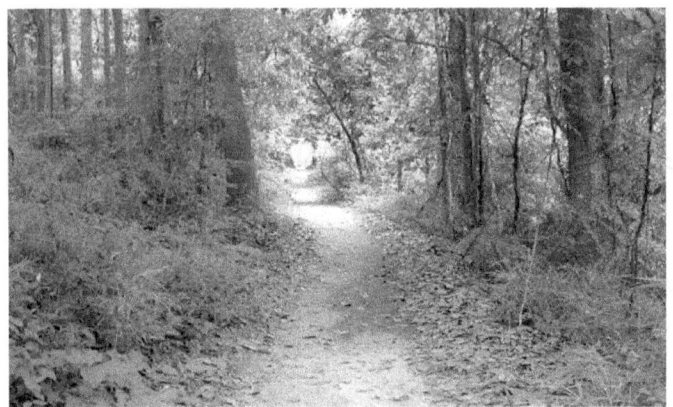

My Personal Journey Through Bariatric Surgery

Bibliography

BMI Chart http://www.bmi-calculator.net/bmi-chart.php

Highland Hospital Bariatric Center. Obtained on 1/11/2013. Retrieved from

Mayo Clinic Obtained on 12/14/14. Retrieved from http://www.mayoclinic.org/bariatric-surgical

St Vincent Carmel Hospital Obtained on 1/10/2013. Retrieved from

St Vincent Bariatric Weight Loss Center of Excellence. Roux-en-y Gastric Bypass Booklet. Obtained 3/7/2013 at preop class for bariatric surgery.